THE ABUNDANCE OF WEALTH THAT HEALTHY LIVING BRINGS

Simple Steps to Achieving a Healthier Life

STEVE ARTHUR

I dedicate this book to all the good People everywhere in the world. Thank you for making the world a beautiful place for all to live peacefully.

THE ABUNDANCE OF WEALTH THAT HEALTHY LIVING BRINGS

Simple Steps to Achieving a Healthier Life

STEVE ARTHUR

ISBN: 9798387460708
Imprint: Independently published

DEDICATION

I dedicate this book to all the good People everywhere in the world. Thank you for making the world a beautiful place for all to live peacefully.

INTRODUCTION

Health and wellness are both essential for our lives. You cannot be successful in anything unless you are healthy!
Staying healthy means taking care of ourselves so that we can live a full life without physical or mental illness.

We all know the importance of our physical health and how it affects our daily lives, but what about its effect on job satisfaction? Studies have shown that employee health has a direct correlation with job satisfaction.

A healthy lifestyle can lead to improved productivity, better performance, and even fewer sick days taken. Not only can investing in your physical health help you perform better at work, but it can also lead to a more positive working environment overall.

After all, if employees are feeling their best mentally and physically they'll be more likely to enjoy their job and be productive while doing it. Investing in your physical health is not only beneficial for yourself but also for those around you—it's a win-win situation!

Crafting a lifestyle based on health and wellness includes eating nutritious foods, exercising regularly, getting enough sleep, managing stress, and socializing with friends and family.

Caring for our bodies comes with a lot of perks, such as elevated energy levels, better moods, improved productivity at work or school activities, lower risk for chronic illnesses like diabetes or hypertension, and a higher quality of life overall. Making small positive changes in our daily lives is an easy way to start forming habits that will lead us to overall health and well-being!

CHAPTER 1

Achieving Greater Mental Wellness: Combating the Low Moods.

Mental health is a crucial component of overall good health and well-being. It involves our emotional, psychological, and social well-being, which can be influenced by a variety of things such as our environment, lifestyle choices, and relationships. Mental health impacts how we think, feel, and act daily; it also affects how we manage stress, connect with others, and make decisions.

Poor mental health may result in various issues like depression, anxiety, or relationship difficulties. On the other hand, good mental health allows us to live life with balance - having the capability to deal with the highs and lows that come with life. That's why it's so important for all of us to take steps towards sustaining good mental health for us to function optimally in our lives.

Depression is a common mental health disorder that can present itself in many forms. Typical symptoms include sustained feelings of sadness, trouble focusing, low energy, lack of enthusiasm, and the inability to enjoy pleasure.

Additional signs to watch for are changes in eating habits or sleeping patterns, difficulty making decisions, and thoughts of hurting oneself or suicide. Everyone's experience with depression is unique and there are many resources for those having mental health issues.

Anxiety is yet another mental health problem that can cause physical sensations like chest pain, heart palpitations, and excessive perspiration as well as psychological symptoms such as unrealistic fears or worries about everyday events.

Those who experience anxiety may find it hard to socialize or take on new tasks since they're afraid of failing or being embarrassed. If one finds themselves dealing with recurrent panic attacks they should seek professional aid right away.

Stress plays a significant role in our overall well-being mentally and physically. While short-term stress often has its advantages when managed appropriately, overlong stress creates both physical fatigue and emotional depletion which affects our ability to cope with daily life; this could lead to burnout if left unabated for too long.

The symptoms linked to stress include annoyance, insomnia/restlessness, increased susceptibility towards sickness/injury plus diminished job output – all elements that need

managing through relaxation methods like yoga/meditation or lifestyle modifications such as dietary/exercise plans, visualization of nature, etc.

Practicing relaxation techniques can bring many positive effects, such as slowing your heart rate and breathing rate, reducing how active stress hormones are, increasing blood flow to major muscles, relieving chronic pain, and improving your focus and mood.

It even helps with improving sleep quality and lowering fatigue! To maximize the benefits of relaxation methods, use them together with other healthy coping strategies such as thinking positively, using humor to solve problems, managing your time effectively, exercising regularly, eating healthily, getting ample sleep, and spending time outdoors. Additionally, don't forget to reach out to your supportive family and friends.

Medication can be used to treat mental health conditions if behavioral therapy alone isn't enough. Depending on the condition, there are many kinds of medications – some work by changing brain chemistry or blocking messages in the nervous system. Though, it's important to talk to a doctor before starting any medication as some come with significant
side effects.

CHAPTER 2

Strengthening Your Mind, Body, and Soul Through Exercise.

Physical health is an important aspect of overall well-being and has numerous benefits for both the body and mind. Regular exercise not only helps to maintain physical strength, but it can also help reduce stress levels, improve mental clarity, and promote emotional stability. Exercise also helps to protect against chronic diseases like heart disease and diabetes while improving sleep quality. Additionally, regular physical activity can boost self-esteem and confidence as well as increase energy levels throughout the day. Overall, taking care of your physical health is essential for living a happier life in every way possible.

One of the most important factors to consider when understanding your physical health is diet. Eating a healthy and balanced diet that consists of lean proteins, whole grains, fruits and vegetables, and low-fat dairy products can help to maintain overall health by providing essential vitamins and minerals for energy production as well as supporting the immune system. Additionally, avoiding processed foods high in saturated fat or added sugars can help reduce the risks of developing chronic diseases such as diabetes or heart disease.

Another factor to consider when assessing your current level of physical health is activity level. Regular exercise helps build muscle strength while also increasing cardiovascular endurance levels. Exercise has numerous benefits including improved sleep quality, reduced stress levels, increased confidence levels, higher energy throughout the day, and protection from chronic illnesses like diabetes or heart disease.
While it's important to stay active every day for optimal well-being, make sure not to overdo it; there should be plenty of rest days included in an exercise routine too!

Lifestyle choices play an important role in determining one's overall physical health status. Habits such as smoking cigarettes or drinking alcohol excessively have been linked with numerous negative consequences on both mental and physical health; quitting these habits can have significant positive impacts on overall well-being.

Rest and Sleep

Rest and sleep are essential for our health and well-being, as both have an important role in maintaining a healthy balance between the physical, mental, and emotional aspects of our lives. Our bodies need rest to repair themselves after periods of activity while sleeping helps support the body's systems such as cardiovascular function, metabolism, and physical healing.

During rest and sleep, many physiological processes take place that help us feel rejuvenated when we wake up. This includes allowing muscles to relax from any tension built up during the day; blood pressure dropping; heart rate slowing down; breathing becoming slower; hormones being regulated which helps maintain appetite control; temperature variations which aid digestion and improve cognitive functions like memory formation. In addition to these benefits, adequate amounts of good quality sleep also impact other aspects such as mood regulation or concentration level.

The amount of rest needed is individualized based on factors like age or lifestyle but generally, adults should get 7-8 hours of uninterrupted sleep per night while children require more due to their growing bodies' needs. Furthermore, experts recommend avoiding screens at least one hour before bedtime so your brain can gradually shut down in order to prepare for a good night's restful slumber.

Creating a good sleep space is an important part of maintaining healthy sleep hygiene. This includes making sure the bedroom is dark, cool, and quiet to create an environment that encourages restful slumber.

If possible, it can be beneficial to remove any electronics from the room such as TVs or phones which may emit blue light that could disrupt the production of melatonin needed for deep sleep cycles. It's also helpful to make sure there are no distractions present such as having your phone next to your bed while you're trying to fall asleep since this could cause unnecessary stress if something like a notification pops up during the night.

Regular exercise is a vital part of maintaining physical and mental health. Working out has many perks such as better cardiovascular health, aiding in weight loss or maintenance, increasing muscle and bone strength, reducing stress levels, promoting sound sleep habits, and giving you more energy throughout the day.

You may opt for conventional activities like running or cycling for cardio; weight lifting for strength training; yoga or Pilates to become more flexible; and balance exercises to promote stability.

Additionally, there are many alternative activities to choose from - from dance classes to rock climbing! Be sure to tailor your activity level to your own needs - some may prefer high-intensity interval training while others may like a slower pace with less intense workouts. Beginners should always warm up before starting any physical activity as well!

The advantages of exercising regularly are plentiful: improved heart health due to increased oxygen flow through the body; increased metabolism leading to burning fat cells faster; improved mental clarity due to endorphins released during exercise; decreased stress levels due to reduced cortisol production (the hormone responsible for feeling stressed); stabilized joints helping you creating healthy movement patterns; and improved mood due to higher self-confidence after achieving workout goals. All these benefits will ultimately keep you healthier in both body and mind.

CHAPTER 3

FRUITS AND VEGETABLES FOR   ATHLETIC PERFORMANCE

When you think of a diet to build muscle, your mind probably turns to these classic options. You will probably focus mainly on protein sources such as chicken,
tuna, and eggs. An athlete's diet should consist of nothing but meta and steamed rice right?
But this is far from the only food useful for building
muscles and improving performance. Bodybuilding, sprinting,
swimming, long-distance running, and any other sporting activity are very important
A balanced diet that includes a wide variety is important
for different food groups. It is especially important to get fruits and vegetables.

Are you interested in taking supplements to improve your athletic performance? what
You might be interested to know that eating fruits and vegetables can be
more powerful while costing much less and having countless other amazing features
health benefits!
Here are some samples. The best fruits and vegetables that heal
Sports activity

Beetroot

Beets are far from the most important vegetable
for muscle building and for all kinds of athletes. This is because beets are one of the most effective foods in the world
and raise nitric oxide. Nitric oxide is a natural "vasodilator". it means
that it can cause blood vessels (veins and arteries) to dilate (dilate).
promotes the flow of oxygen and nutrients in the body.
The result is that the muscles receive more oxygen and energy during exercise and
more nutrients to speed recovery. This can help you lift more reps and run longer distances and recover faster.

Spinach

Spinach is a vegetable that is high in protein as well as being a good source of
phytoecdysteroids. These don't have anything in common with anabolic
steroids
but they may have a similar effect
– with some studies suggesting they are a good option for encouraging
muscle building and testosterone production.

Kale

Kale is the vegetable highest in calcium. Calcium is very important for
your workouts, not only does it help to strengthen the bones but it also
reinforces
your connective tissue and it helps to strengthen contractions for more
explosive
power during workouts.
Kale is very trendy right now being high in protein and low in calories. A shame
it
costs a fair bit though!

Mushrooms

Mushrooms are technically not fruits or vegetables, but they are found in the
same aisle and they're safe for vegans, so they're fair game to include here.
Mushrooms are not only another great source of protein but also come with a
wide range of additional health benefits and advantages. They're packed with
minerals, they can encourage recovery from training, and much more besides!
It's surely only a matter of time until we start seeing mushroom protein shakes
cropping up in health stores!
The other amazing benefit of mushrooms is that they contain vitamin D. In fact,
they're one of the few dietary sources of vitamin D! (Another being oily fish).
This is important seeing as vitamin D is considered to be a master hormone
regulator, and is responsible for encouraging the production of testosterone in
particular – one of the main anabolic hormones for building muscle and
burning
fat.
What's more, is that vitamin D has recently been shown to be much more potent
than even vitamin C when it comes to supporting the immune system and
preventing colds and flu. As any athlete knows, a cold can be enough to
complete derail and athletes' training plan, which in turn can be the difference

between victory and failure!

Apples

Apples are rich in vitamin C, which is another crucial vitamin for enhancing the immune system and helping athletes train longer and harder without fail. Vitamin C also helps to encourage the repair of muscle tissue, and increases serotonin to aid with mental recovery, and even increase the production of both testosterone and nitric oxide when paired with zinc.
On top of all this, apples are also very rich in fiber, which can help to improve bowel movements, the absorption of food, blood pressure, and more. Fiber is also key to supporting a healthy microbiome, which in turn can support a healthy
immune system, better mood, weight loss, and much more.

Potatoes

Carbohydrates are often maligned, but they are a lot
important for muscle building and physical training in general. Potatoes have a good choice of carbohydrates as they are also high in fiber and vitamin C (which improves recovery) and low in calories. Use after training and
the energy goes directly to the muscles of the waist.

Carrots

Carrots are generally healthy and a great source of vitamins A, C, and K. What's exciting about them though is the lutein, which may help to increase energy levels and enhance the efficiency of your very mitochondria!
Your mitochondria are the energy factories of your cells which convert glucose into ATP (glucose being the sugar that comes from carbs, and ATP being the usable form of energy in your body). This in short means that with carrots and other sources of lutein, you can run faster and you'll burn
more calories even when you're resting!
In one study, rats were given lutein (which needs a source of fat to absorb such as
milk) and it was found that they began running long distances voluntarily in their
wheel, burning much more fat than they did.

Wonderful Fruits And Vegetables For Mood, Energy, Beauty And More

oh, you are not very interested in losing weight? Maybe you are already
satisfied with your size? (Good for you!)
Maybe you're not an athlete? You may not have remarkable health
problems. See, fruits and vegetables are good for everyone. And just to drive that
point home,
here are more examples of fruits and vegetables that have
various health benefits.

**Broccoli and Leafy Greens for Beauty
and Pregnancy**
Yes, fruits and vegetables can help to make you look more beautiful. And that's
true even of something as simple as your humble broccoli!
Broccoli is perhaps a little less 'exotic' when compared with some of the other
superfood fruits and vegetables on this list. But don't let that fool you: this is
still
an incredibly nutritious food that everyone should be getting more of.
For starters, broccoli is a good source of fiber and can once again help to improve
your digestion, your bowel movements, and much more. On top of that though,
broccoli is also very high in vitamins K, vitamin C, fiber, potassium, collagen,
iron,
calcium, and more.

Let's start by diving into that collagen. This is something that all of us need but
very few of us get it. Collagen has been shown to improve brain function and
combat against Alzheimer's, it also helps to reduce back pain, improves skin
elasticity strengthens the nails, combats leaky gut syndrome, fights knee pain,
and generally toughens up your tendons, ligaments, and bones.
This is why meals such as bone broth as so incredibly good for us. And now
recent
research is suggesting an even more powerful reason that collagen might be so
important. Researchers now suspect that humans would once have lived
primarily
by eating bone marrow from animal carcasses.

The argument goes that hunter-
gatherers may have been ill-equipped to take on large prey. However, we were
very good at tracking down our prey and following them.
What likely would have happened often, is that we would have followed
antelopes and other animals to the point where they were attacked and killed by
animals like lions and tigers. They would then have stripped those animals of all

their meat, leaving behind the skeleton. That's when the cunning and resourceful
humans would have come along, broken open the bones with our tactile hands, and then eaten the nutritious collagen from inside.

If this is indeed true, then we evolved in an environment where we consumed large amounts of the constituents of bone. And we now find ourselves flung into a
world where we very rarely get these crucial nutrients. If that's the case, then broccoli may be even more beneficial than we first assumed!

Pregnant mothers should look into eating more broccoli and more
greens in general. That's because both broccoli and many salad leaves are good sources of folate, which is something that all mothers are recommended to eat. Not getting enough folate increases the risk of complications in pregnancy, and that's why a lot of mothers will try and get more artificially through the use of pregnancy supplements.

This is where it's important to point out the significant advantages of getting more nutrients from your diet rather than from supplements. While it's true that
you can benefit from supplements, the clue here is in the name.

These are intended to supplement your regular diet.
That is to say that they should be taken in addition to your regular diet, rather than as an alternative. Nutrients from your diet are far more effective than those
taken in pill form, as they are combined with numerous other nutrients, fats, fibers, and other elements.

Together, these help to improve absorption of the key elements and that makes them much more effective. The thing to recognize is that the human body evolved while being exposed to these foods and therefore is optimally designed to extract the nutritional value in this form.
It is not designed to consume nutrients in a synthetic form. This is why so many tell you not to take vitamin tablets on an 'empty stomach'. They just work better as food.

Cayenne Pepper for Weight Loss, Testosterone, and More
Cayenne pepper meanwhile is another great tool in the battle against inflammation. This is a compound that makes food spicy and is widely found in ointments and creams due to its anti-inflammation effects. It's a common pain-

relief too as it depletes nerve cells of the chemical 'substance P'. Substance P causes both inflammation and the sensation of pain, so this is a great thing to add to your diet if you do suffer from a condition like fibromyalgia or arthritis. Cayenne also comes packed with flavonoids and carotenoids.

These are
antioxidants that prevent cellular damage, thereby further combating against inflammation.
Cayenne pepper also has several other impressive benefits. It has been shown to be an effective appetite suppressant, for instance, meaning that if you are someone who struggles to stick to a diet, you might start finding it a little easier to be disciplined and thereby hopefully see the weight begin to fall off. At the same time, cayenne pepper may help to improve digestion. This is important because better digestion doesn't only give you more energy and prevent discomfort, but it also helps you to better absorb nutrients from your food. That means that all the benefits you're getting from the other superfoods on this list will then be turned up to 11.
What's more, is that cayenne pepper has also been shown to increase testosterone. This of course is the hormone that most of us know as the 'male hormone' and is responsible for the male sex drive, as well as many of the differences between men and women. Increasing testosterone in men increases muscle tone, reduces fat storage, raises aggression, aids with recovery, fortifies the immune system, and more.

Men who don't get enough testosterone will exhibit signs of depression, low energy, low mood, and low sex drive. They also struggle with weight gain and low
muscle mass. Conversely, men with high testosterone exhibit the traits that we associate with the classic 'alpha male' along with toned and powerful physiques. This is why so many men try to augment their natural testosterone production through the use of steroids and other drugs – despite those carrying numerous health warnings and serious dangers.
The worrying part is that testosterone in men is increasing across the globe by 1% a year. This is partly due to the use of feminine products and their impact on our water, along with a host of other problems (certain plastics and our generally inactive lifestyles). But diet plays a BIG part in it too. Time to start eating
a little less processed food, and a little more cayenne pepper.

Elderberry for Inflammation

Elderberry is a berry that is rich in nutrients. It is once again a fruit that is absent
from many of our regular diets, so it's one that you should consider reintroducing.
The simple fact of the matter is that most of us rely on the same few fruits and vegetables day in and day out. This way though, we are ensuring we get a lot of nutrients in effect while missing out on some others. The best diet is the most varied diet – the one that includes the biggest range of different fruits, vegetables, meats, herbs, and more. So what can elderberry do for you?
Elderberry has been used since prehistoric times and has been used as a supplement or medicine by a host of ancient cultures – including the Ancient Egyptians. Today we now know that these fruits are incredibly high in flavonoids
and anthocyanins.

At the same time, elderberries have been shown to help boost the production of cytokines. These are the messenger molecules that our bodies use in order to control the immune system. Pro-inflammatory cytokines help to encourage inflammation, while anti-inflammatory cytokines help to reduce them. This is all
very important because it ensures that the body is able to properly
regulate its response to viruses and diseases and to help heal wounds and injuries.
Many of us think that inflammation is always a bad thing – though,
inflammation helps to destroy infections before they have a chance to take effect,
as well as to encourage healing by delivering more nutrients to the affected area.
The problem is when this response goes haywire.
It turns out that for similar reasons, elderberry might also be highly
effective at combating allergies!
On top of all this, elderberries are also highly effective at combating and destroying pathogens, being useful in fighting infections, colds, and a host of other problems. Most interesting of all, the tiny berries contain potent antiviral agents that have been shown to actually 'deactivate' viruses.
These work by preventing the viruses from being able to break through cell walls
using their haemagglutinin spikes, which in turn renders them almost inert. They
are thus very effective for combating problems like rhinitis, as well as preventing

them from occurring in the first place.
Of course, there is also the usual vitamin and mineral content that you tend to get from berries.

CHAPTER 4

Exploring the Causes and Effects of Pollution on Our Health.

Pollution is the introduction of contaminants into our environment that cause harm and disruption to the natural balance. Pollutants can be both man-made or naturally occurring, but all have an adverse effect on our health and the environment.

The most common causes of pollution include air pollution from vehicles, agricultural activities such as burning fossil fuels and chemicals used in fertilizers, and water contamination due to industrial runoff.

Types of pollutants include particulate matter (PM), carbon dioxide (CO), nitrogen oxides (NOx), and sulfur dioxide (SO).

And other hazardous materials are released into the atmosphere by various sources like factories, power plants, construction sites, etc.
These pollutants are not only detrimental to human health but also lead to global warming which further has a devastating impact on ecosystems around us.

Water Pollution: We are seeing more and more of our water sources becoming contaminated by substances like fertilizers, pesticides, and animal waste, which can be poisonous when ingested by humans through either drinking contaminated water or eating food grown near polluted sources.

Sewage overflows can also lead to the growth of bacteria that causes serious illnesses like cholera and typhoid fever. To help stop this issue from getting worse, we need better monitoring systems in place to detect contamination quickly while enacting stricter regulations on the disposal of hazardous materials into waterways.

Soil Quality: Human-induced deforestation practices over the past years have severely depleted the soil's nutrient content necessary for healthy vegetation growth, leading to major soil erosion and poorer crop yields depending on location and climate conditions. Long-term solutions include restoring soil fertility through more effective farming techniques such as no-till agriculture which helps maintain topsoil quality.

Respiratory Health: Air pollution is one of the biggest threats to respiratory health, as it can lead to a range of issues including asthma, bronchitis, and other chronic obstructive pulmonary diseases (COPD).
Particulate matter from vehicle emissions and industrial smoke is particularly dangerous when inhaled because they contain dangerous particles that can easily enter our lungs and cause harm to the body system.

To reduce the risk here we need to invest in cleaner-burning fuels for vehicles and switch over to alternative energy sources like solar power; improve ventilation systems in buildings; phase out high-emission equipment or manufacturing processes; reduce the burning of wood or coal for cooking or heating; avoid aerosol sprays indoors etc.

Cardiovascular Health: In addition to air pollution, environmental factors such as water contamination can also have an impact on cardiovascular health due to toxins found in contaminated water which can cause inflammation leading to stroke, heart attack, and other adverse outcomes.

To protect against this we need improved monitoring systems that detect contamination early, so measures can be taken quickly before it spreads too far into the environment.
Also, stricter regulations regarding the disposal of hazardous waste materials into waterways should help reduce future instances of water contamination significantly.

Cancer: Environmental pollutants have been linked with various types of cancer such as lung cancer caused by prolonged exposure to tobacco smoke or chemical carcinogens like asbestos fibers which lodge deep within the lungs when inhaled causing serious damage over time leading to even death if left untreated. To mitigate these risks

Health Effects of Pollution
Effects on Human Health: Pollution can cause a range of health issues in humans, from respiratory problems to heart disease and cancer. Inhaling polluted air has been linked to asthma, bronchitis, COPD (Chronic Obstructive Pulmonary Disease), emphysema, lung cancer, and other illnesses that affect the cardiovascular system.

Long-term exposure to pollutants such as smog or ground-level ozone can also lead to premature death due to lung damage caused by free radicals generated from chemical reactions with pollutants in the atmosphere.

Effects on Plants and Animals: Pollutants in the environment can have devastating effects on plants and animals living nearby. Many aquatic species are especially vulnerable since they rely so heavily on clean water for survival; toxic chemicals like mercury or DDT which get into waterways can bioaccumulate up through the food chain leading to serious health impacts for fish, birds, and other wildlife who ingest them at high concentrations. Air pollution may also reduce plant productivity and increase their susceptibility to disease due to changes in soil chemistry caused by acid rain.

Effects on Natural Ecosystems: As pollution accumulates over time it slowly begins altering natural ecosystems; these changes can be very difficult if not impossible to reverse depending upon how much damage has been done already.

Effects include habitat destruction due to disruption of food webs as well as direct mortality resulting from contact with hazardous materials released into the environment such as oil spills or nuclear radiation leaks. This is why it's important for us all to take action against pollution now before irreversible harm is done!

Environmental health is a critical issue that must be addressed to protect human health and the environment. Improving environmental health requires us to take action both individually and collectively to reduce pollution, conserve resources, and mitigate the impact of climate change.

We can start by making conscious choices about our energy usage such as using renewable sources like solar power or wind turbines; reducing water consumption; avoiding single-use plastics where possible; properly disposing of hazardous materials like paint thinners or pesticides etc.

At the same time, we need governments around the world to enforce stricter regulations on industries polluting the environment for their financial gain while also investing more in research and development of alternative energy sources. Ultimately improving environmental health will require a collective effort from everyone to create a healthier planet for future generations.

Government must enforce strict standards on what products are allowed into the marketplace as well as encourage individuals to take precautions such as avoiding smoking cigarettes or using insulation containing asbestos fibers if possible.

Preventing Pollution

Environmental Laws and Regulations: As a society, we must all do our part to prevent pollution by following the laws and regulations set in place. These laws and regulations are designed to protect both human health as well as natural ecosystems from the devastating effects of pollution. For example, many countries have banned or regulated certain chemicals or emissions known to be hazardous for human health and/or nature, such as leaded gasoline or chlorofluorocarbons (CFCs). Likewise, governments can also enact legislation intended to limit air pollution from industrial sources like power plants which often release an excessive amount of pollutants into the atmosphere.

Reduce, Reuse, Recycle: One of the most effective ways to mitigate future environmental damage is through responsible consumption habits with regards to resources; this means reducing our use of single-use items whenever possible while also reusing whatever we can so that it doesn't end up in landfills where it will eventually break down releasing pollutants into nearby soil & water supplies. Additionally making sure we recycle whatever materials we consume responsibly will ensure they don't end up becoming waste that needs disposal either!

CHAPTER 5

How to Unlock Your Inner Strength and Harness Positive Emotions.

Emotional health is the ability to recognize, express, and manage our emotions in a healthy way. It involves developing an understanding of how we feel and why, as well as learning how to effectively communicate those feelings with others. In addition to managing stress levels, cultivating emotional health helps us build strong relationships and strengthens our resilience against life's challenges.

As an individual attending to one's emotional well-being is essential for leading a fulfilled life. Taking the time to check in with our feelings and address any anxieties can be beneficial in creating a state of contentment.

Understanding emotion begins with understanding the power of emotions. Emotions are an integral part of our daily lives as they guide our decisions, allow us to express ourselves, and make life meaningful.

The brain is responsible for processing emotions, and it does this by using a complex network of neurotransmitters that communicate between different areas in the brain. These systems affect how we feel about things, how we respond to situations, and even how we think or behave.

Emotional responses can be conscious or unconscious, allowing us to process information quickly while still being aware of what is happening around us. For example, when something positive happens you may experience feelings such as happiness or joy while if something negative happens your body responds with fear or sadness.

Understanding these reactions helps you recognize them in yourself as well as others so that you can work towards better managing your emotional health and responding appropriately to difficult situations in relationships or other social settings.

It's also important to understand that emotions don't always come from external sources; internal factors such as stress levels or mental health issues can contribute significantly to emotional states too.

When faced with these challenges it's essential to take care of oneself by engaging in activities like exercise, and relaxation techniques like creating art as an outlet for dealing with emotions,
creating art, viewing it, and talking about it provide a way for people to cope with emotional conflicts and increase self-confidence.

Talking through problems with friends/family/therapists, etc., all of which have been proven effective at improving emotional well-being over time.

Stress is an unavoidable part of living, but by understanding and dealing with it, we can help to ensure our emotional health. When exposed to a stressor, the body releases hormones like cortisol and adrenaline, sparking the 'fight or flight' response which was designed to be a protective measure.

Unfortunately, when this response is triggered too often due to chronic pressures of life, it can lead to serious mental distress.

Chronic stress can impair our ability to regulate emotions and can result in mental disorders like anxiety or depression if not managed carefully. Physically too, it takes its toll on the body; increasing heart rate and blood pressure, weakening the immune system, and making us prone to illnesses.

Above all else though, it stops us from enjoying life since we are always worrying about potential disadvantages instead of focusing on activities that will lead to overall well-being.

It's essential that we recognize when we are feeling overwhelmed by stress so that we can fight it before our mental health is affected too severely.

Taking time out of each day for activities such as physical exercise, meditation or reading may reduce levels of stress as well as leading to healthier reactions which won't worsen our condition in the future. Furthermore, seeking professional help via counseling sessions or support groups is invaluable for those struggling with extended periods of anxiousness/depression caused by long-term pressure on their psychological
state.

CHAPTER 6

Practicing Healthy Habits: Easily Incorporate into Your Everyday Life.

Stay hydrated

We all know how simple it is to seize another can of pop or cup of coffee rather than another glass of water. With the wide cluster of beverages available these days, water continuously appears just like a boring choice.

It's always so easy to opt for a can of soda or a cup of coffee rather than taking the time to fill up your water bottle. But, keep in mind that your body needs water to get your brain functioning, help circulate blood, and regulate your body temperature. Plus, we're constantly losing water throughout the day - whether it's due to breathing, sweating, or using the restroom. So, you must remember to stay hydrated!

Here are the tips for remaining hydrated:

- Know how much water you would like to expend each day

- Make drinking a glass of water part of your normal routine

- Carry a water bottle

- Try unsweetened sparkling water or flavor your water by adding fresh fruits, vegetables, and herbs
- Track your water intake using an app
- Choose hydrating snacks, such as cucumbers, celery, strawberries, or watermelon
- Distribute your water intake throughout the day (playing catch up at the end of the day doesn't negate the fact that you were dehydrated all day.

When you stick to a diet of nutrient-rich foods, it's beneficial for your overall mental health. Studies have found that eating mainly whole, unprocessed foods can help with symptoms of depression and anxiety. So, what should you be putting in your cart at the grocery store? Here's a quick overview!

Whole foods

It's important to stay away from preservatives, food colorings, and additives that may worsen hyperactivity and depression. Instead, focus on real food or food that's minimally processed and has a few healthy ingredients. Colorful fruits and vegetables contain powerful nutrients that have tons of benefits for the mind and body due to their nutritional properties contained in the colors themselves.

The science behind food and mood

There is a connection between nutrition and emotions that comes from the close relationship between your brain and your gastrointestinal tract (also known as the "second brain").

The bacteria in your gut influence the production of certain hormones such as serotonin which are then sent by chemical substances to the brain; when production is optimal our mental state will be reflected positively. Too much sugar however, can feed "bad" bacteria in the gut, resulting in short-term pleasure followed by an unwelcome crash afterward.

Fiber, antioxidants, folate, vitamin D, and magnesium are other key elements when it comes to considering food for our mental health. Plant-based foods are full of fiber which helps regulate glucose levels; berries, leafy green vegetables, and spice turmeric contain antioxidants; folate is found in leafy greens, lentils, and cantaloupes; mushrooms are another good source of vitamin D; magnesium is essential for nerve and muscle function but can also be found in cacao nibs, almonds, cashews, spinach and dark leafy greens, bananas, and beans; finally fermented foods are packed with probiotics which are key for digestive tract health.

And don't forget about being present while eating! Noticing how your food smells, tastes, and feels can help you combat cravings or overeating.

A diet rich in fruits and vegetables has important health benefits, including weight control and reduced risk of many chronic diseases. The reality is that if you don't eat enough fruits and vegetables, you're missing out on the health benefits they provide.

It also may mean you're filling up on calorie-dense foods or ones that are heavily processed — which, when eaten in excess, can come with health disadvantages.

Eating whole and unprocessed foods is an important part of creating a healthy diet. This means eating food as close to its natural state as possible and avoiding pre-packaged snacks or meals that are high in added sugar, salt, and fat.

Eating a variety of different types of food can also help you get the essential vitamins and minerals your body needs for optimal health. Fruits, vegetables, lean meats, legumes, and dairy products are all examples of nutritious foods that should be included in your daily diet.

Limiting processed and refined food can also go a long way towards improving your overall well-being. These highly processed items often contain unhealthy levels of salt and fat which can lead to weight gain or other chronic health issues if consumed regularly. Additionally, they tend to lack nutritional value, so it's best to stick with fresh produce instead whenever possible.

Finally, making sure you drink enough water each day is key for keeping your body hydrated which helps maintain proper bodily functions such as digestion, circulation, and temperature regulation. Drinking at least 8 glasses per day will ensure your body has the fluids it needs to perform optimally throughout the day!

CHAPTER 7

Understanding the Urgency of Climate Change and Global Warming

Climate change and global warming are two of the most pressing environmental issues facing our planet. They refer to an increase in average surface temperatures caused by rising levels of greenhouse gases, primarily from human activities such as burning fossil fuels and deforestation.

This leads to a disruption in the Earth's climate system, resulting in extreme weather events, droughts, floods, heatwaves, and sea level rise - all factors that threaten natural ecosystems around the world.

The effects of climate change are already being felt across the globe; Arctic ice is melting faster than ever before while coral reefs have been bleached due to higher ocean temperature levels. We must take action now to mitigate these impacts if we want a better future for ourselves and generations to come.

Natural Causes of Climate Change and Global Warming

The Milankovitch cycles, also known as orbital variations, are a fundamental driver of climate change. These alterations to the Earth's orbit lead to changes in solar radiation received at different latitudes, resulting in significant long-term shifts over thousands of years. The most recent cycle began approximately 20, 000 years ago and is still ongoing today. This natural phenomenon leads to global warming seen over the past century due to increased temperatures from incoming solar radiation.

Volcanic eruptions can have both short-term and long-term effects on climate change, depending on their size and composition. A major eruption can inject large amounts of aerosols into the atmosphere which reflect sunlight away from the Earth's surface leading to cooling temperatures for several months or even up to two years afterward.

The 1991 eruption of Mt Pinatubo is an example where average global temperatures decreased by
5 degrees Celsius for three consecutive years following the event - highlighting how powerful these events can be in changing our planet's temperature balance!

Mount Pinatubo's eruption demonstrated the power of these events in impacting the Earth's temperatures, as it caused global average temperatures to drop by 5°C for three consecutive years. El Niños and La Niñas are also important in influencing global climate, as they affect the transport of heat across the Pacific Ocean. El Niños produce more rainfall in South America but can cause droughts elsewhere (e.g., Indonesia). On the other hand, La Niña can bring increased precipitation to North America, but more arid conditions to Australia - showing that this interaction between ocean circulation and climate is quite complex!

Human Factors that Drive Climate Change and Global Warming

Burning fossil fuels releases carbon dioxide which traps heat in the atmosphere creating global warming and climate change. Industrialization began during the 19th century and has caused an unprecedented rise in global temperatures.

Deforestation removes trees, which are natural carbon sinks, resulting in higher levels of global warming. Illegal activities such as poaching or illicit charcoal production can lead to further losses to our planet's health. Human-generated aerosols from sources such as vehicles, industry smokestacks, and wildfires can change cloud formation and albedo, leading to further environmental degradation if unchecked!

Consequences of Climate Change and Global Warming

The consequences of climate change and global warming are far-reaching, affecting virtually all aspects of life on Earth. One of the most visible effects is an increase in average global temperature due to rising levels of greenhouse gases such as carbon dioxide. This has a host of implications, including melting sea ice and glaciers which leads to a rise in sea level that threatens coastal areas around the world. As temperatures continue to climb, habitats are shifting with species being forced into new regions or facing extinction; already many plants and animals have been affected by these changes, while ocean acidification caused by higher concentrations of CO_2 also disrupts delicate marine ecosystems.

These environmental impacts come with economic costs as well; from agricultural losses due to droughts or floods causing food shortages to resource management issues stemming from reduced water availability or disruption in fisheries for example. Furthermore, infrastructure damage resulting from increasingly severe weather events can strain both regional and national budgets further compounding our financial woes!

In addition, there are significant public health risks associated with climate change such as increasing air pollution leading to more respiratory diseases like asthma; vector-borne illnesses like malaria spreading into new areas where they were previously rare; heat waves bringing about deadly heat stroke cases; worsening allergies due warmer temperatures promoting pollen growth – just to name a few examples! This is an issue we must address urgently if we want future generations to be able to enjoy the same quality of life that we do today.

Solutions to Mitigate Climate Change and Global Warming

One of the most effective solutions to mitigate climate change and global warming is to decarbonize our energy sector. This involves transitioning away from fossil fuels as a source of electricity towards renewable sources such as solar, wind, hydroelectricity, geothermal, and bioenergy. Reducing reliance on dirty energy sources like coal and oil can significantly reduce carbon emissions while also providing cheaper and more reliable power for communities around the world. Investment in research & development into new low-cost clean technologies is essential if we are to achieve this goal successfully in the near future!

Conservation and protection of natural ecosystems are another important strategies for fighting climate change. Forests act as vital 'carbon sinks' by absorbing CO2 from the atmosphere; however, deforestation releases these stored carbon molecules back into our air leading to further increases in global temperatures – making it essential that we protect these areas wherever possible! Sustainable agricultural practices such as no-till farming techniques which help keep soil healthy also play an important role here by preventing erosion or nutrient runoff which could otherwise damage fragile habitats downstream.

Finally addressing population growth should be seen as part of any plan attempting to tackle climate change & global warming since higher human numbers mean increased demand for resources (such as food or fuel) all leading towards greater environmental degradation due to overconsumption – something humanity must strive to avoid! Education within local communities on best practices when it comes to water usage, waste management, etc., can go a long way in helping spread awareness about responsible behavior that benefits everybody involved - not just now but well into the future too!

To conclude, it is essential that we take swift and decisive action to tackle climate change and global warming in order to ensure a better future for ourselves and generations to come. We must transition away from fossil fuels towards renewable sources of energy while protecting natural ecosystems, investing in research & development into low-cost clean technologies, and educating communities on best practices related to resource conservation.

Furthermore, population growth should be addressed as part of any comprehensive strategy since overconsumption exacerbates the already dire situation further. With commitment, collaboration, and dedication on our part, we can make sure the planet remains livable for many years to come!

CHAPTER 8

Prioritizing Personal Health: The Right Way to Practice Good Hygiene.

Good hygiene involves the habits that help keep the body and environment clean and free from germs, bacteria, and other contaminants. Practicing good hygiene can reduce the chances of getting ill or infected, improving physical health by preventing illnesses such as colds, flu, or skin infections. Furthermore, taking care of oneself with appropriate personal grooming practices and staying aware of one's surroundings are key components for sustaining excellent hygiene habits throughout life. Good hygiene has psychological advantages too; it boosts self-esteem and encourages a sense of well-being which can lead to better mental health.

The Role of Handwashing:

Handwashing is one of the most important habits for maintaining good personal hygiene. It helps remove potentially infectious bacteria and other contaminants from our hands and prevents them from spreading to others or entering our bodies, thus reducing the risk of illnesses such as colds, flu, and foodborne diseases. Proper handwashing techniques should be taught at an early age in order to ensure that everyone understands how it works effectively. This includes using soap and warm running water for at least 20 seconds before drying completely with a clean towel or air-dryer.

Skin Care and Grooming:

Skin care is another important component of personal hygiene, as it helps keep skin healthy by preventing infections while also promoting a more attractive appearance. Daily cleansing with mild soap can help remove oils and dirt buildup on the surface without causing irritation or dryness; moisturizing afterward will help protect against environmental damage such as windburn or sunburn. Additionally, regular grooming activities like shaving, trimming nails, flossing teeth, brushing hair, etc., are essential for keeping up appearances whilst removing any potential dirt accumulation in those areas which may cause health problems if left unchecked.

Environmental Hygiene

Environmental hygiene is a very important part of staying healthy. Cleanliness and air quality are two major factors that contribute to keeping our environment safe for living.
Improving the cleanliness in our homes can help reduce the risk of illness, allergies, respiratory problems, and even radon poisoning from poor indoor air quality.

The first step in maintaining environmental hygiene is to keep all surfaces free of dirt and dust which may contain bacteria or allergens that could cause harm if inhaled or ingested. Regularly wiping down countertops, floors, furniture, and other surfaces with an appropriate cleaner will help get rid of any potential contaminants while also removing built-up grime or grease which can be breeding grounds for disease-causing organisms. Additionally, it's important to regularly vacuum carpets or upholstered furniture as they tend to trap more dust than hardwood floors do; this should be done at least once a week with a high-efficiency particulate air (HEPA) filter-equipped vacuum cleaner as these have been proven to remove 99% of particles

3 microns in size including pollen, pet dander, mold spores, etc.

Improving home air quality by controlling pollutants within the home such as cigarette smoke has also been found effective in reducing health risks associated with indoor pollution exposure; smoking should therefore not be allowed indoors if possible but rather outdoors away from open doors and windows so that no secondhand smoke seeps back into the house. Other sources like chemical fumes from household cleaners should also be avoided wherever possible due to their potential toxicity levels; using natural solutions made out of common items like vinegar or baking soda instead can help reduce chemical exposure while still allowing you to maintain a clean home without sacrificing your health! Lastly investing in an efficient ventilation system is another key factor when it comes to improving overall air quality within the home – this ensures proper circulation between fresh outdoor air coming in through exhaust fans/windows combined with filtered recirculated stale indoor air being pushed out

Impact of Good Oral Hygiene

Good oral hygiene is essential for maintaining overall health and well-being. Regular brushing and flossing are important for preventing tooth decay, gum disease, bad breath, and other oral health issues. Brushing should be carried out at least twice a day with a soft-bristled toothbrush and fluoride toothpaste to help remove plaque buildup on the teeth's surface. Flossing regularly will also help remove food particles from between the teeth that may cause bacteria growth if left unchecked. Additionally, checking for any signs of oral diseases such as cavities or gingivitis can be done easily by performing regular self-exams or visiting a dentist every six months for professional examinations.

Certain lifestyle choices can also have an impact on our dental health. Quitting smoking or using tobacco products is one of the most effective ways to improve oral hygiene; these substances contain chemicals that can damage both the enamel and gum tissue leading to an increased risk of cavities, periodontal disease, discoloration of teeth, etc. Reducing sugar intake is another key factor in reducing cavity formation while eating foods rich in calcium like dairy products helps strengthen bones which support healthy gums surrounding the teeth. Lastly drinking plenty of water throughout the day helps keep saliva production up which plays an important role in washing away harmful bacteria within our mouths keeping it clean throughout each day!

Conclusion

It's so easy to overlook the importance of our health, but it affects so many facets of our lives. Trying to get back what we took for granted can be a challenge; have you ever tried to lose weight? Much harder than it was to gain it!

That's why it's essential to take steps towards improving your health if you want to be successful. Working out, eating healthily, and making sure that your family does too, are all important. Plus, try not to get overwhelmed; learn how to ask for help when you need it and let go of any baggage that may be weighing you down.

Once you've done this, you will feel rejuvenated - as though years have been knocked off your age - and ready for the life you've always dreamed of. So thank you for reading and here's to good health, happiness, and success!

About Author

The life story of this prolific writer is truly inspiring because it showcases how ambition can take you places regardless of your starting point in life or where you come from. His success is a testament not only to his immense talent but also to his hard work over the years that has enabled him to become who he is today – a celebrated author whose works have been read by millions around the globe.

The writer took steps to establish connections with publishers and industry professionals, attend conferences and pitch ideas, and write for newspapers

33

ABOUT THE AUTHOR

Steve Arthur

The life story of this prolific writer is truly inspiring because it showcases how ambition can take you places regardless of your starting point in life or where you come from. His success is a testament not only to his immense talent but also to his hard work over the years that has enabled him to become who he is today – a celebrated author whose works have been read by millions around the globe.
The writer took steps to establish connections with publishers and industry professionals, attend conferences and pitch ideas, and write for newspapers